Healing Together

A Gentle Guide for Navigating Birth Trauma as a Couple

By Clarinda Brandão

You Are Not Alone: Beginning the Journey

Welcome.

I'm so glad you've found this guide. If you're here, it's likely because you or someone you love has experienced birth trauma. First, let me say this: you are not alone. Birth trauma can be an overwhelming and isolating experience, leaving you with questions, pain, and perhaps even a sense of disconnect from yourself or your partner. But there is hope. This guide is designed to be a supportive companion on your journey to healing - a way to process, understand, and move forward with compassion and intention.

I'm a therapist who has spent many years working with individuals and couples navigating the aftermath of birth trauma. In my practice, I've witnessed the profound impact that trauma can have - not just on the birthing person, but on their partner and the relationship as a whole. I've seen how trauma can challenge even the strongest partnerships, creating emotional distance, communication breakdowns, and struggles with intimacy. But I've also seen how couples and individuals can emerge from this experience stronger, more connected, and more resilient than ever before.

Some of the couples I've worked with came to me feeling lost and unsure of how to navigate the changes brought on by trauma. The birthing person may have been carrying the weight of physical pain, emotional exhaustion, or feelings of inadequacy, while their partner struggled with helplessness, guilt, or their own version of trauma. In some cases, the trauma created unspoken tensions, while in others, it led to outright conflict. Each story was unique, yet a common thread ran through them all: a desire to heal, to reconnect, and to find hope on the other side.

For individuals, birth trauma can feel like a deeply personal wound - one that's hard to explain or share with others. I've worked with people who felt ashamed of their pain or believed they should just "get over it." Through our work together, we explored how trauma is not a sign of weakness but a natural response to an overwhelming experience. With time, they learned to process their emotions, reclaim their sense of self, and embrace the idea that healing is possible.

This guide is the culmination of what I've learned through years of supporting people just like you. It's a blend of professional insight, practical tools, and heartfelt empathy. My hope is that as you move through these chapters, you'll feel seen, understood, and empowered to take the steps that feel right for you and your unique journey.

Before we begin, I want to acknowledge the courage it takes to face trauma and commit to healing. This is not an easy path, but it's one worth walking. Whether you're here as the birthing person, the partner, or both, this guide is for you. It's a space to explore your feelings, strengthen your relationship, and find the tools you need to rebuild and reconnect.

As you dive into this guide, give yourself permission to take it at your own pace. Healing is not a race - it's a process that unfolds gradually, one step at a time. Be gentle with yourself and your partner as you move through the exercises and reflections. Some sections may resonate deeply, while others may feel challenging.

That's okay. There is no right or wrong way to use this guide; it's here to support you, wherever you are in your journey.

My work has taught me that trauma can transform us in ways we never imagined. It can open the door to deeper understanding, stronger connections, and profound resilience. This guide is not just about surviving birth trauma - it's about finding hope, healing, and the strength to thrive together.
Let's take this step forward, together.

Warmly,
Clarinda

Chapter 1
Understanding Birth Trauma

What is Birth Trauma?

Birth trauma refers to the physical and emotional distress experienced during childbirth, which can significantly impact both the birthing person and their partner. It's not just about physical injury or medical complications - it's also about how the birthing experience is perceived. When the experience is overwhelming, frightening, or leaves one feeling helpless or unsafe, it can result in lasting emotional and psychological effects.

Emotional vs. Physical Trauma

- **Physical Trauma:** This could involve complications such as a long labor, emergency interventions like a C-section, or unexpected medical challenges for the birthing person or the baby.
- **Emotional Trauma:** Even when physical outcomes are positive, emotional trauma can arise when the birth does not go as expected, leaving a person feeling powerless, unheard, or out of control.

Both physical and emotional aspects are equally important, and trauma may manifest differently in the birthing person and their partner.

The Role of Expectations and Control

A key element of birth trauma is the disconnect between expectations and reality. Often, parents go into childbirth with a certain plan or ideal, but when things take a turn - be it medical complications, lack of communication from healthcare providers, or unexpected outcomes - feelings of disappointment, fear, or betrayal can surface. Losing a sense of control during childbirth is a significant factor in birth trauma.

How Birth Trauma Impacts the Birthing Person

For the person who physically experiences childbirth, birth trauma can manifest as:

- Intense fear during the process of labor or delivery
- Feelings of powerlessness or helplessness
- Emotional disconnect from the experience, leading to numbness or shock
- Guilt or shame if the birth didn't go as planned or they feel they didn't "perform" as expected

How Birth Trauma Affects Partners

While the birthing person is often the focus of trauma discussions, partners can also experience their own version of birth trauma, sometimes referred to as **secondary trauma**. Partners may feel:

- Helplessness as they watch their loved one in distress, unable to intervene
- Anxiety or fear for the health and safety of both the birthing person and the baby
- Guilt for not being able to protect or support their partner in the way they envisioned
- Emotional shock from unexpected complications or outcomes

Why Understanding Trauma Matters

Recognizing that birth trauma affects both individuals is critical to healing as a couple. Both the birthing person and the partner need to understand that these emotions and reactions are valid. By acknowledging the trauma - whether it was physical, emotional, or both - you can begin to take steps toward recovery, individually and together.

In the coming chapters, we'll explore how this trauma can affect your relationship, your roles as new parents, and the healing process both of you need to navigate. It's important to remember that trauma isn't about what *should* have happened, but rather about how the experience was *felt* by both of you. Healing starts with understanding.

*****

Exercise: Sharing Your Birth Experience

This exercise is designed to help both the birthing person and their partner share their feelings and experiences in a safe, supportive environment. The goal is to foster understanding and empathy between partners as you begin to process the trauma together.

Step 1: Set the Scene

- Choose a time when you both can be fully present - away from distractions like phones, children, or work.
- Find a quiet, comfortable space where you can talk without interruptions. Make sure both of you feel emotionally prepared to have this conversation.
- Bring a notebook or journal, as well as something to drink, like tea or water, to create a calming environment.

Step 2: Reflect Individually

Take 5-10 minutes to individually reflect on your birth experience. Write down your thoughts in a notebook or journal. Answer the following questions:

- For the birthing person: What moments during the birth stand out most in your memory? How did you feel during the experience - physically and emotionally? What expectations did you have for the birth, and how did reality differ?
- For the partner: What were the most intense moments for you during the birth? How did you feel watching your partner go through the experience? What fears, anxieties, or hopes did you have before, during, or after the birth?

Step 3: Share Your Experiences

- Once you've both had time to reflect, take turns sharing your responses.
- When one person is speaking, the other should practice active listening. This means:
    - No interrupting.
    - Listening without judgment or trying to "fix" the other person's feelings.
    - Acknowledging the other's emotions with simple responses like "I understand," or "That sounds really hard."

Step 4: Ask Questions for Understanding

After each person has shared, take turns asking questions to better understand your partner's experience:

- For the partner: "What was the hardest part for you?" or "What do you wish I had known or understood during the birth?"
- For the birthing person: "What do you need from me now?" or "How can I support you in healing?"

Step 5: Validate Each Other's Feelings

- Affirm that both of your feelings are valid. It's okay if you had different experiences or reactions to the same event. Trauma affects people in unique ways.
- Say something supportive to your partner, such as "I'm so sorry you went through that," or "I'm here for you, no matter what."

Step 6: Close with a Moment of Connection

- End the exercise by spending a quiet moment together. This could be a hug, holding hands, or simply sitting in silence, acknowledging that you're facing this healing journey as a team.
- Take a deep breath together and express gratitude for one another.

Reflect Together

After the exercise, consider these reflection questions:

- What surprised you about your partner's experience or feelings?
- How can you both continue to support each other in the healing process?
- What do you need to feel more connected moving forward?

Chapter 2
Recognizing the Signs of Trauma

The Subtle and Not-So-Subtle Signs of Trauma

Trauma manifests differently in every person, and its symptoms can be physical, emotional, or behavioural. Recognizing these signs in yourself or your partner is the first step toward healing. This chapter will help you identify how trauma may be showing up in your lives, even if it isn't immediately obvious.

For the Birthing Person

Common signs of trauma may include:

Emotional Symptoms:

- Persistent feelings of fear, sadness, or anger
- Numbness or emotional detachment
- Intrusive thoughts or flashbacks about the birth experience
- Avoidance of reminders of the birth (e.g., avoiding talking about it or visiting the hospital)

Physical Symptoms:

- Difficulty sleeping or nightmares
- Physical tension or chronic pain, particularly in the pelvic or abdominal areas
- Fatigue or feeling physically drained

Behavioral Symptoms:

- Increased irritability or frustration
- Difficulty bonding with the baby or withdrawing from loved ones
- Reluctance to seek help or talk about the experience

For the Partner

Partners can also experience trauma, even if they weren't the one giving birth. Signs of trauma in partners may include:

Emotional Symptoms:

- Helplessness or guilt for not being able to protect their partner during the birth
- Anxiety about the baby's or partner's well-being
- Resentment or frustration about the experience

Physical Symptoms:

- Insomnia or restlessness
- Fatigue or exhaustion from emotional and physical stress

Behavioural Symptoms:

- Withdrawal from the birthing person, baby, or social connections
- Increased irritability or difficulty managing stress
- Overcompensating in caregiving roles to regain a sense of control

How Trauma Can Affect Your Relationship

Trauma doesn't just impact individuals - it also affects your partnership. Some common relationship challenges include:

- Difficulty communicating: Both partners may struggle to share their feelings openly, leading to misunderstandings.
- Emotional disconnection: One or both partners might feel distant or isolated, even in the same space.
- Changes in intimacy: Physical closeness may feel overwhelming or unattainable after trauma.

Understanding these signs can help you recognize when it's time to seek support, either from each other or from a professional.

***

Exercise: Identifying Trauma's Impact

This exercise helps you and your partner reflect on how trauma is showing up for each of you and in your relationship.

Step 1: Reflect Individually

Take 5 minutes to answer the following questions in a notebook or journal:

- What changes have I noticed in myself since the birth experience? (Emotionally, physically, behaviorally)
- What changes have I noticed in my partner since the birth?
- How do I think trauma has impacted our relationship?

Step 2: Share with Your Partner

Once you've reflected, share your answers with each other. Remember:

- Use "I" statements, such as "I feel..." or "I've noticed..." to avoid placing blame.
- Be patient and listen without interrupting.

Step 3: Create a Joint List

Together, create a list of the specific ways trauma has impacted your relationship. For example:

- "We don't talk as much as we used to."
- "I feel anxious when I think about the birth."
- "We've been avoiding intimacy."

Step 4: Identify a Small Step Forward

Choose one area from your list where you can take a small, positive step together. For example:

- If communication is a challenge, commit to a weekly check-in to talk about feelings.
- If intimacy feels distant, start with small gestures of physical closeness, like holding hands.

By recognizing the signs of trauma and how it affects both of you, you can begin to understand that these experiences are valid and normal. Naming these challenges is the first step toward addressing them as a team. The next chapter will focus on how birth trauma impacts parenting and your new family dynamic.

Chapter 3
The Impact on Relationships

Trauma and Connection: The Hidden Ripple Effect

Birth trauma doesn't just affect individuals - it ripples outward, impacting relationships in profound ways. For many couples, the experience challenges the foundation of their partnership. Feelings of disconnection, miscommunication, or resentment can arise, often leaving both partners feeling isolated and misunderstood.

This chapter explores how birth trauma affects intimacy, communication, and partnership dynamics, providing insights to help couples navigate these challenges together.

Common Relationship Challenges After Birth Trauma

Emotional Disconnection

- The birthing person may withdraw due to feelings of guilt, shame, or fear.
- The partner may feel helpless, unsure how to provide support, or resentful if their efforts seem unnoticed.
- Both may experience emotional numbness, making it hard to connect.

Communication Breakdowns

- Trauma often silences honest conversations. The birthing person may avoid discussing the experience, while the partner might not know how to bring it up.
- Misunderstandings arise when emotions are left unspoken, leading to assumptions or blame.

Intimacy Challenges

- Physical closeness, including sex, may feel overwhelming for the birthing person, especially if the trauma involved their body.
- The partner may misinterpret this as rejection, further straining the relationship.

Parenting Tensions

- Birth trauma can magnify differences in parenting styles or expectations, creating conflict where there was once harmony.

Why It Can Happen

Birth trauma significantly impacts relationships because it disrupts the emotional and physical equilibrium partners share. This disruption often stems from the differing ways each person experiences the trauma. For the birthing person, the trauma is intensely physical and emotional, involving their body and a profound sense of vulnerability. For the partner, the trauma is often experienced from a place of helplessness, as they watch their loved one endure pain and fear without being able to intervene effectively. These unshared experiences create a gap in understanding, as neither partner can fully grasp what the other went through, leaving both feeling isolated in their pain.

Emotional dysregulation is another way trauma affects relationships. Trauma disrupts the brain's ability to process emotions effectively, leading to heightened states of anxiety, sadness, or irritability. This emotional upheaval can manifest as impatience, withdrawal, or frustration, often unintentionally hurting the other partner. Without tools to manage these emotions, couples can find themselves stuck in patterns of miscommunication or avoidance, further widening the emotional gap between them.

Unspoken expectations also contribute to the strain. Both partners may enter the postpartum period with differing assumptions about recovery and support. For example, the birthing person may expect their partner to intuitively know how to support them emotionally, while the partner may assume that once the physical wounds heal, things will return to normal. When these expectations are unmet, frustration and resentment can build, as neither feels fully understood or supported.

The shift in roles after childbirth adds yet another layer of complexity. Even under normal circumstances, becoming parents is a monumental adjustment. With trauma in the mix, these new roles can feel overwhelming. The birthing person may struggle with feelings of inadequacy as a parent due to lingering trauma or physical recovery, while the partner may feel an increased burden to "hold everything together," leaving little room to process their own emotions.

Intimacy, both physical and emotional, often takes a backseat after trauma. The birthing person may feel disconnected from their body, viewing it as a source of pain rather than pleasure. This can make physical closeness feel overwhelming or even frightening. For the partner, this withdrawal can feel like rejection, even if it's not intended that way. The loss of intimacy, coupled with the emotional disconnection trauma often brings, can make it difficult for couples to feel close in any meaningful way.

Understanding why these challenges arise is essential for both partners to approach each other with empathy and patience. Trauma is not about fault or weakness; it's a natural response to an overwhelming experience. Recognizing these dynamics as part of the healing journey, rather than as signs of failure, is the first step toward rebuilding your connection.

Reconnecting as a Couple

Healing as a couple after birth trauma requires intentional effort to rebuild trust, communication, and intimacy. It begins with empathy - the ability to step into your partner's shoes and understand their perspective. Trauma often creates a divide, as each partner processes the experience in their own way. For the birthing person, this might mean grappling with feelings of powerlessness or fear, while the partner might struggle with helplessness or guilt. Acknowledging these feelings and validating each other's experiences is the foundation of reconnection. For example, the birthing person might say, "I know it must have been hard for you to watch me go through that without being able to help," while the partner might express, "I can't imagine how scary that must have been for you, and I wish I could have done more."

Open communication is another vital step. Trauma often silences couples, as it can be difficult to put overwhelming emotions into words. However, healing starts with honest dialogue. Setting aside regular times to check in with each other can create a safe space to talk about your emotions. Active listening - where each partner reflects back what the other has shared - can help avoid misunderstandings and ensure both feel heard. It's important to use "I" statements, such as "I feel disconnected" or "I'm struggling with intimacy," rather than assigning blame. This approach fosters understanding and reduces defensiveness.

Rebuilding trust is essential after trauma, as it can sometimes feel fragile or shaken. Small, consistent actions are key. Being reliable - keeping promises, being present, and showing up emotionally - can go a long way in demonstrating commitment to the relationship. Patience is equally important, especially when it comes to vulnerability or physical intimacy. Trust grows when both partners feel safe and supported in expressing their needs and fears without judgment.

Physical intimacy can feel daunting after trauma, especially for the birthing person. Reintroducing closeness gradually and without pressure is an effective way to rebuild that connection. Start with small, non-sexual gestures like holding hands, hugging, or sitting close together. These acts of affection can help reestablish a sense of safety and connection. It's important for the birthing person to feel in control of their body and for the partner to respect their boundaries. Offering reassurance, such as saying, "I'm here for you whenever you feel ready," can create a nurturing environment for intimacy to return at its own pace.

Creating new rituals as a couple can also help restore stability and connection. Trauma often makes life feel unpredictable, so small, intentional rituals can provide comfort and structure. This could be as simple as sharing a morning coffee, taking a short walk together, or ending the day by expressing gratitude for each other. These consistent, positive interactions can strengthen the bond between you and remind you of your shared commitment.

Finally, it's important to acknowledge the positives in your relationship, even amidst the challenges of healing. Trauma can be an opportunity for growth, as it often reveals the depth of your resilience and the strength of your partnership. Take time to celebrate the ways you've supported each other, whether through small acts of kindness or simply being there during difficult moments. Reminding yourselves of the love and dedication you share can provide hope and motivation to continue working on your connection.

Reconnecting after birth trauma is a journey, not a destination. It requires patience, vulnerability, and mutual effort. There will be good days and tough days, but each small step toward understanding and supporting each other strengthens your relationship. Healing doesn't mean forgetting the trauma - it means learning how to move forward together, with love and resilience.

***

Exercise: Mapping Your Relationship's Emotional Terrain

This exercise helps you and your partner identify areas where your relationship has been impacted by birth trauma, opening a pathway to understanding and reconnection.

Step 1: Reflect Individually

Take 5-10 minutes to write down answers to the following questions:

- How has the birth experience changed the way I feel about myself?
- How has it changed the way I feel about my partner?
- What do I miss most about our relationship before the birth?

Step 2: Share Your Answers

Take turns sharing your reflections. Use "I feel…" or "I've noticed…" statements to keep the focus on your experience rather than assigning blame.

Step 3: Identify Your Shared Pain Points

Together, identify specific ways your relationship has been affected. Examples might include:

- Difficulty talking about feelings.
- Avoidance of physical intimacy.
- Increased conflict about parenting roles.

Step 4: Set an Intention for Reconnection

Choose one small, actionable step to reconnect. Examples:

- Commit to a weekly check-in conversation about your emotions.
- Reintroduce small gestures of affection, like hugs or holding hands.
- Plan a short "date" at home, even if it's just 10 minutes of uninterrupted time together.

Building a Foundation for Healing

Understanding that trauma is not your fault—and that it's possible to rebuild—is key to healing your relationship. By taking small steps toward vulnerability, empathy, and connection, you can begin to strengthen your partnership.

The next chapter will delve deeper into coping strategies for both partners, providing tools for individual and shared healing.

Chapter 4
Coping Mechanisms and Healing

The Path to Healing

Healing after birth trauma is a deeply personal and collaborative process. It requires each partner to explore their individual experiences while supporting one another in recovery. Coping mechanisms and healing strategies can empower both partners to regain a sense of stability and connection, fostering emotional resilience and creating space for growth.

Coping Mechanisms for the Birthing Person

The birthing person often carries the physical and emotional scars of trauma. Coping mechanisms for healing focus on rebuilding trust in their body and processing their emotions:

Reclaiming Your Body: Trauma can leave you feeling disconnected from your body. Practices such as gentle yoga, meditation, or body scans can help rebuild this connection. Start by acknowledging and honoring what your body has endured.

Expressing Emotions: Journaling, art, or talking with a trusted friend or therapist can provide an outlet for emotions that feel overwhelming.

Practicing Self-Compassion: Remind yourself that your trauma does not define you, and healing takes time. Celebrate small victories and progress, even if it feels incremental.

Coping Mechanisms for the Partner

Partners often face their own version of trauma, grappling with feelings of helplessness, guilt, or secondary trauma. Their healing process requires attention to their emotional needs:

Processing Your Emotions: It's normal to feel a range of emotions, from anger to sadness. Finding ways to process these - through therapy, journaling, or physical activity - can help alleviate the burden.

Supporting Without Overextending: While being a source of support for your partner is important, it's equally vital to care for yourself. Setting boundaries and taking time to recharge will make you more effective in your role.

Finding a Peer Support Network: Connecting with other partners who have experienced birth trauma can provide a sense of solidarity and understanding.

Coping Together

Healing as a couple is about navigating the trauma as a team. It's not just about recovering individually but also about strengthening your partnership:

Setting Shared Goals: Discuss what healing looks like for both of you. Is it feeling more connected? Rebuilding physical intimacy? Creating shared goals can give you a roadmap.

Practicing Patience: Healing is not linear, and each partner may progress at a different pace. Be patient with each other and recognize that setbacks are part of the process.

Engaging in Joint Activities: Spend time doing things you both enjoy. Whether it's cooking, walking, or watching a favorite show, these moments can help rebuild your connection.

***

Exercise: Building Your Coping Toolkit

This exercise is designed to help each partner identify and implement coping strategies that resonate with them.

Step 1: Reflect on What Helps You Cope

Take 5 minutes to individually brainstorm a list of activities, behaviors, or habits that have helped you cope with stress or challenges in the past. Examples might include:

- Physical activities (e.g., walking, yoga, exercise)
- Creative outlets (e.g., painting, writing, music)
- Social support (e.g., talking to a friend, joining a support group, therapy)
- Relaxation techniques (e.g., deep breathing, meditation, baths)

Step 2: Share Your Lists

Take turns sharing your lists with your partner. Discuss:

- What strategies have worked well for you in the past?
- What could you try together to support healing?

Step 3: Create a Joint Toolkit

Together, create a list of coping mechanisms you can try individually and as a couple. For example:

- Individual: Journaling, therapy, or mindfulness exercises
- As a couple: Walking together, sharing a daily check-in, or practicing gratitude

Step 4: Commit to Trying One New Strategy

Choose one coping mechanism from your joint list to implement this week. Reflect on how it felt and whether it helped strengthen your sense of well-being or connection.

Healing is a Journey

Healing from birth trauma is a deeply personal process that unfolds differently for everyone, and it's rarely a straightforward path. It's not a simple matter of moving on or forgetting the experience; rather, healing involves learning how to live with the trauma, making sense of it, and finding ways to move forward with resilience. It's important to recognize that there will be ups and downs - moments of progress followed by setbacks. These fluctuations are a natural part of the process and do not mean that healing is out of reach. Trauma is not something that can simply be erased, but its impact can lessen over time as you work toward understanding and integration.

Each partner will have their own timeline for healing, and that's okay. The birthing person may need to focus on physical recovery and emotional processing simultaneously, while the partner may be dealing with feelings of helplessness, guilt, or secondary trauma. These different timelines can sometimes feel frustrating, but they're a reminder that healing is not a one-size-fits-all process. Patience and compassion for both yourself and your partner are key to navigating this journey together. Understanding that you may be in different places emotionally allows you to better support one another without judgment.

It's easy to focus on the big picture and wish for immediate resolution, but healing is often found in the small, consistent steps you take together. Moments like holding hands, sharing a quiet conversation, or simply sitting in silence can create a sense of connection that helps rebuild your emotional foundation. These small acts of care and kindness toward yourself and your partner are not insignificant - they are the foundation of recovery. Celebrating these moments, no matter how small, reinforces the progress you are making.

Trauma has the potential to change people, but it doesn't have to define your life or your relationship. Many couples who face birth trauma together find that it can serve as a catalyst for growth. It's not about forgetting the pain, but rather about learning from it and using it as a source of strength and understanding. By working through the trauma together, you can develop deeper empathy for one another, greater emotional resilience, and a stronger bond as partners and parents.

Finding meaning in the healing process can also be a powerful tool. This doesn't mean justifying the trauma or believing that everything happens for a reason, but instead asking, "What can we take from this experience?" For some, the answer may be developing a greater appreciation for their relationship, learning to advocate for themselves and others, or simply growing more attuned to each other's needs. These insights can help reframe the trauma as something that, while painful, also contributed to your growth as a couple.

Support plays a vital role in the healing journey. You don't have to go through this process alone. Whether it's through therapy, support groups, or trusted loved ones, reaching out for help can ease the burden of recovery. Support provides perspective, validates your experiences, and reminds you that you're not alone. Couples who seek support together often find that sharing vulnerability in a safe space strengthens their relationship and helps them navigate the healing process more effectively.

As time goes on, you may begin to reflect on the trauma with less intensity. The memories will likely still exist, but they can lose their power to overwhelm you. Looking back at how far you've come - both individually and as a couple - can be incredibly affirming. This reflection helps you see your resilience and growth, paving the way for a future filled with hope and possibility.

Ultimately, healing is a shared commitment. It's about showing up for one another, even when it's hard, and embracing the process with patience and love. It's a promise to not only survive the trauma but to thrive beyond it, finding strength in your partnership and building a foundation for the future. The journey may be challenging, but it's also an opportunity to rediscover yourselves and each other in ways that can bring you closer than ever before.

Chapter 5:
Navigating the Medical System

Advocating for Your Care

After a traumatic birth experience, navigating the medical system can feel overwhelming. The healthcare environment that once represented hope and safety may now bring anxiety or frustration. However, understanding how to advocate for your care and for your partner's - can be an empowering step toward healing. This chapter focuses on how to engage with medical professionals, ask the right questions, and ensure both partners receive the support they need.

Understanding Post-Trauma Medical Needs

Birth trauma can leave lingering physical and emotional scars that require attention. For the birthing person, this might involve addressing physical injuries such as perineal tears, cesarean scars, or pelvic floor dysfunction. Emotional scars like anxiety, depression, or post-traumatic stress disorder (PTSD) also need professional care. Partners may also require emotional support for secondary trauma or the stress of caregiving. Acknowledging these needs is the first step in seeking effective care.

Many people delay follow-up care after birth trauma, either because they feel overwhelmed or because their trauma has caused mistrust in the medical system. It's important to recognize that healthcare providers can be valuable allies when approached with clear communication and boundaries. By preparing ahead of time and knowing what to ask, you can reclaim a sense of control over your care.

Preparing for Medical Appointments

Preparation can make medical appointments feel less daunting. Here are some tips to make the most of these visits:

Write Down Your Concerns

- Make a list of physical and emotional symptoms you've experienced since the birth. Include anything that feels significant, even if you're unsure whether it's related to the trauma.
- Partners should also prepare notes about their own concerns or observations, as these can provide valuable insights to healthcare providers.

Be Specific About Your Needs

- If you're seeking help for physical recovery, ask for referrals to specialists like pelvic floor physiotherapists or pain management clinics.
- For emotional recovery, inquire about counseling services, support groups, or trauma-informed mental health professionals.

Prepare Questions

Examples of helpful questions include:

- "What options are available for treating this issue?"
- "Can you refer me to someone who specializes in trauma recovery?"
- "What resources are available for partners or families?"

Advocating During Appointments

It's common to feel vulnerable during medical appointments, especially after trauma. Advocacy is about ensuring your voice is heard and your needs are met. Here's how to approach it:

Be Honest About Your Experience

- Share what happened during the birth and how it has affected you. Use clear, specific language to describe your physical and emotional symptoms.

Ask for Trauma-Informed Care

- Trauma-informed care involves providers who understand the impact of trauma and approach treatment with sensitivity. Don't hesitate to request a provider who practices this approach.

Bring a Support Person

- Having your partner or another trusted individual present can help you feel more supported and ensure that all your concerns are addressed.

Supporting Each Other's Medical Needs

Partners play a crucial role in navigating the medical system together. Here's how to work as a team:

For the Partner:

- Attend appointments whenever possible to provide emotional support and help your partner remember important details.
- Advocate on their behalf if they feel overwhelmed or struggle to express their concerns.

For the Birthing Person:

- Encourage your partner to seek care for their emotional well-being, especially if they've experienced secondary trauma.

Supporting each other through this process reinforces your connection and shows that you're tackling the healing journey as a team.

*****

Exercise: Crafting Your Advocacy Plan

This exercise helps you and your partner prepare for medical appointments and advocate effectively for your care.

Step 1: Identify Your Needs

Each of you should take a few minutes to reflect on the following questions:

- What physical or emotional challenges am I currently facing?
- What do I want to achieve by seeking medical care?
- What fears or anxieties do I have about interacting with healthcare providers?

Step 2: Create a List of Priorities

Together, write down a list of the most pressing concerns for each partner. Rank them in order of importance to ensure nothing gets overlooked during appointments.

Step 3: Develop Questions for Providers

Based on your priorities, create a set of questions to ask healthcare providers. Examples might include:

- "What treatments or therapies do you recommend for this condition?"

- "What resources are available to help us cope with trauma?"
- "How can we access mental health support for both partners?"

Step 4: Role-Play Advocacy

Practice how you'll approach the conversation with your provider. One person can play the role of the healthcare professional while the other practices expressing their concerns and asking questions. Switch roles to build confidence.

Reclaiming Control

Navigating the medical system after birth trauma is not just about addressing physical injuries or emotional scars—it's about reclaiming a sense of control over your well-being. By preparing for appointments, advocating for trauma-informed care, and supporting each other, you can turn a daunting process into an empowering step forward. Remember, seeking help is not a sign of weakness but an act of courage and self-care.

In the next chapter, we'll discuss how trauma impacts parenting and explore ways to balance healing with the challenges of caring for a new baby.

Chapter 6
Parenting After Trauma

The Challenges of Parenting After Trauma

Parenting a newborn is a demanding journey for any couple, but when birth trauma is part of the experience, those demands can feel even heavier. Trauma impacts how you approach caregiving, bond with your baby, and manage the stress of parenting. It's not uncommon for both the birthing person and their partner to feel conflicted - grateful for their baby yet overwhelmed by lingering fears, anxieties, or physical challenges.

This chapter explores the unique challenges of parenting after trauma and provides tools to help you navigate this transformative time while prioritizing healing and connection as a family.

The Birthing Person's Experience

For the birthing person, physical recovery often overlaps with the emotional work of processing trauma. This can complicate their ability to engage fully in caregiving, leaving them feeling guilty or inadequate. They might:

- Struggle with bonding due to feelings of disconnection or fear of failing as a parent.
- Experience anxiety about their baby's health or safety, sometimes stemming from medical complications during birth.
- Feel physical limitations from injuries, making everyday caregiving tasks exhausting or painful.

It's important to remember that these feelings and challenges are valid. Healing takes time, and there is no "right" way to parent after trauma.

The Partner's Experience

For partners, the transition into parenting can be equally complex. Partners may:

- Feel unsure of their role, especially if they are trying to shield the birthing person from additional stress while managing their own emotions.
- Struggle with secondary trauma or feelings of helplessness from the birth experience, which may interfere with bonding with the baby.
- Feel pressure to "keep it all together," leading to emotional burnout or frustration.

Acknowledging these challenges and seeking support can help partners feel more confident and connected in their parenting role.

The Impact on Bonding

Bonding with your baby is a central part of parenting, but trauma can create obstacles. The birthing person might feel emotionally detached, while the partner might worry about doing things "right." These feelings are normal, but they can improve with intentional efforts to connect with your baby:

- Spend time holding, cuddling, or making eye contact with your baby, even if it feels awkward at first.
- Engage in skin-to-skin contact, which can help regulate both your baby's and your emotions.
- Take turns caring for the baby so both partners have opportunities to bond.

Building a connection with your baby doesn't have to be instant. It's okay if the bond develops gradually over time.

Managing Parenting Stress

Parenting is stressful under the best circumstances, and trauma can amplify those stresses. Coping strategies can help you manage this stress together:

> **Prioritize Rest:** Fatigue can make everything feel harder. Work together to establish a sleep schedule that allows each of you some uninterrupted rest.

> **Simplify Expectations:** Focus on what's truly important and let go of unnecessary tasks. It's okay if the laundry piles up or the house isn't spotless.

> **Share Responsibilities:** Divide caregiving tasks so that neither partner feels overwhelmed. This also helps ensure both of you have time to focus on self-care.

> **Communicate Regularly:** Check in with each other about how you're feeling and what support you need. Even a few minutes of honest conversation can make a big difference.

Balancing Parenting and Healing

It's easy to feel like you have to choose between being a good parent and focusing on your recovery, but the truth is, both can coexist. Taking care of yourself allows you to show up for your baby and partner in a more meaningful way. Consider these tips:

For the Birthing Person:

- Be patient with yourself. Your baby doesn't need perfection - they need love and care, which you are already providing.

- Seek professional help for physical recovery or emotional trauma if needed.

For the Partner:

- Recognize your value in the parenting role, even if it feels secondary at times.
- Practice self-care to prevent burnout and maintain emotional balance.

***

Exercise: Building a Parenting Plan

This exercise helps couples manage the challenges of parenting after trauma by creating a plan that prioritizes both caregiving and healing.

Step 1: Identify Each Partner's Strengths

Take a moment to reflect on what each of you feels confident about when it comes to parenting. For example:

- The birthing person might feel good about feeding or soothing the baby.
- The partner might excel at diaper changes or nighttime routines.

Write down these strengths to build a sense of shared confidence.

Step 2: Divide Responsibilities

Discuss and write out a rough plan for caregiving tasks. Examples:

- Who will handle feedings, diaper changes, or nighttime care?
- How can you share household chores to lighten the load for both partners?

Step 3: Incorporate Self-Care

Each partner should identify one self-care activity they want to prioritize, whether it's taking a walk, meditating, or simply having quiet time. Discuss how to support each other in carving out time for these activities.

Step 4: Plan Check-Ins

Commit to regular check-ins, even if they're brief. Use this time to talk about how you're feeling, any adjustments needed to the plan, and what's working well.

A Family Journey

Parenting after trauma is not without its challenges, but it also offers an opportunity for immense growth and connection. The early days of parenting may feel overwhelming, particularly as you navigate the dual paths of caregiving and healing. However, it's important to remember that these two processes are not mutually exclusive. In fact, they often complement each other. As you work to heal, you're also building the emotional and physical capacity to care for your baby, and as you nurture your baby, you may find moments of joy and connection that contribute to your healing.

While the journey may be difficult, it is also deeply rewarding. Every small step you take - whether it's comforting your baby during a sleepless night, sharing a meaningful moment with your partner, or acknowledging your own progress - is a testament to your resilience as a family. These moments, though they may feel small in the moment, are the building blocks of a stronger family foundation.

Parenting after trauma also offers a chance to redefine your family dynamics. By consciously addressing the challenges of trauma, you can create a family environment that prioritizes empathy, understanding, and connection. Your shared experiences of overcoming adversity can foster a deeper sense of closeness, as you learn to rely on and support one another in new ways. Over time, these shared efforts can strengthen not only your relationship with your partner but also the bond you both share with your child.

It's important to embrace the idea that there's no one "right" way to parent after trauma. Your journey may look different from others, and that's okay. What matters most is that you approach this process with patience and compassion for yourselves and each other. Healing doesn't require perfection - it requires showing up each day with love, intention, and a willingness to grow together.

Ultimately, parenting after trauma is a journey of transformation. It's a chance to rebuild not only yourselves as individuals but also your relationship as partners and your connection as a family. While the path may be uncertain, it's filled with opportunities to create a nurturing, supportive environment where both healing and love can flourish. By embracing this journey, you are giving your family the greatest gift: a foundation of resilience, understanding, and unwavering care.

Chapter 7
Communication & Support Between Partners

The Foundation of Connection

Birth trauma can create barriers in communication, leaving partners feeling isolated in their struggles. The overwhelming emotions and stress of trauma often lead to silence, avoidance, or misunderstandings. However, open communication and mutual support are essential for healing, both as individuals and as a couple. This chapter focuses on practical strategies to rebuild communication, express needs, and strengthen your partnership as you navigate the aftermath of trauma together.

Why Communication Breaks Down After Trauma

Trauma can disrupt communication in subtle yet significant ways. For the birthing person, feelings of guilt, shame, or fear may make it difficult to share their emotions. They might worry about being a burden to their partner or fear that their pain won't be understood. Partners, on the other hand, may avoid bringing up their own struggles, believing that their role is to support rather than to share. This can lead to both individuals bottling up their feelings, creating emotional distance.

Additionally, misunderstandings often arise when trauma affects how each partner interprets or reacts to situations. One partner may see withdrawal as a sign of rejection, while the other views it as self-protection. Without open dialogue, these assumptions can lead to conflict or resentment. Rebuilding communication requires patience, empathy, and a willingness to step into each other's shoes.

Practical Communication Strategies

Reestablishing communication takes effort and intentionality. Here are strategies to help you and your partner reconnect through honest, empathetic dialogue:

Create a Safe Space

- Set aside regular times to check in with each other in a calm, distraction-free environment.
- Approach conversations with the intention to listen and understand, rather than to fix or defend.

Use "I" Statements

Express your feelings in a way that focuses on your own experience, rather than blaming or accusing. For example:

- "I feel disconnected when we don't talk about how we're feeling."
- "I'm struggling to know how to support you, and I'd like to understand what you need."

Practice Active Listening

When your partner speaks, reflect back what you hear to ensure understanding. For example:

- It sounds like you're saying you feel overwhelmed. Is that right?"
- Avoid interrupting or jumping to conclusions, and resist the urge to offer solutions unless your partner asks for them.

Validate Each Other's Feelings

Acknowledge that both of your emotions are valid, even if they differ. Saying something like, "I can see why that would make you feel anxious," helps your partner feel heard and understood.

Be Patient with Silence

Not every conversation will flow easily, especially when discussing difficult topics. Allow space for pauses and give your partner time to process their thoughts.

How to Offer Support

Support isn't always about solving problems—it's about being present and showing your partner that they're not alone. Here's how to provide meaningful support:

Ask, Don't Assume

Instead of guessing what your partner needs, ask directly:

- "How can I support you right now?"
- "What do you need most from me today?"

Be Attuned to Nonverbal Cues

Sometimes, your partner's body language can tell you more than their words. Pay attention to signs of stress, exhaustion, or sadness, and respond with small acts of care, like offering a hug or taking over a task they're struggling with.

Respect Boundaries

Everyone processes trauma differently. If your partner needs space, respect that boundary while letting them know you're there when they're ready to talk.

Offer Reassurance

Remind your partner that you're in this together. Simple affirmations like, "We'll get through this as a team," or,

"You're doing an amazing job," can provide comfort and encouragement.

*****

Exercise: Rebuilding Connection Through Conversation

This exercise is designed to help you and your partner reconnect by practicing intentional communication.

Step 1: Share One Thing You're Feeling

Each partner takes turns sharing one thing they've been feeling lately - good, bad, or neutral. Be specific and use "I" statements. For example:

- "I've been feeling anxious about how we're handling everything."
- "I've felt grateful for how you've been supporting me."

Step 2: Reflect Back What You Heard

After one partner shares, the other reflects back what they heard. For example:

- "It sounds like you're feeling anxious because there's so much happening right now."

Step 3: Respond with Empathy

The listening partner responds with empathy, avoiding solutions unless asked. For example:

- "I can understand why you feel that way. That sounds really tough."

Step 4: Switch Roles

Repeat the process with the other partner sharing their feelings.

Step 5: End with Gratitude

Close the conversation by expressing gratitude for each other's openness. For example:

- "Thank you for sharing that with me. I really appreciate how honest you were."

Building a Stronger Partnership

Rebuilding communication and support after trauma is not about getting it perfect every time - it's about showing up with intention and care. Each conversation, no matter how small, is a step toward understanding and connection. The goal is to create a partnership where both of you feel safe to share, supported in your struggles, and confident in your ability to face challenges together.
Strong communication lays the groundwork for deeper intimacy and a more resilient relationship. In the next chapter, we'll explore the benefits of seeking professional help and how therapy can provide additional tools to support your healing journey as a couple.

Chapter 8
Seeking Professional Help

Why Therapy Matters

Healing from birth trauma is a challenging journey, and while many couples can make significant progress on their own, professional help can provide the tools, guidance, and safe space needed to navigate the complexities of trauma and its impact on your relationship. Therapy allows both partners to process their individual experiences, improve communication, and rebuild intimacy under the guidance of a trained professional. This chapter explores the benefits of therapy, when to seek it, and what to expect from the process.

When to Consider Therapy

It's not always easy to know when professional help is needed. Therapy can be especially beneficial if you or your partner are experiencing:

- Persistent emotional or physical symptoms of trauma that interfere with daily life.
- Difficulty discussing the birth experience or related feelings with each other.
- Ongoing feelings of guilt, shame, or blame within the relationship.
- Struggles with bonding with your baby or adapting to new parenting roles.
- Challenges with intimacy or unresolved conflicts.

Even if your symptoms don't feel "severe," therapy can be a proactive step toward strengthening your relationship and addressing the impact of trauma.

Types of Therapy

There are several therapeutic approaches that can support couples navigating birth trauma. Understanding these options can help you choose what's right for your situation:

Trauma-Focused Therapy

- Designed to help individuals process and reframe traumatic experiences.
- Examples: Eye Movement Desensitization and Reprocessing (EMDR), somatic therapy, Talk Therapy with a Trauma-Informed Therapist, or cognitive processing therapy.

Couples Therapy

- Focuses on improving communication, resolving conflicts, and rebuilding intimacy between partners.
- Often incorporates trauma-informed approaches to address the impact of trauma on the relationship.

Individual Therapy

- Provides a safe space for each partner to work through their own emotions and challenges.
- Can complement couples therapy by addressing personal struggles that may affect the partnership.

Parenting-Focused Therapy

- Helps couples navigate the challenges of parenting after trauma, focusing on bonding with the baby and managing parental stress.

What to Expect in Therapy

Starting therapy can feel intimidating, but understanding what to expect can make the process more approachable:

The First Session
During your initial therapy session, the focus will be on creating a safe and supportive environment where you feel comfortable sharing your experiences at your own pace. Your therapist will likely begin by asking general questions about your birth experience, the challenges you've been facing, and what you hope to achieve through therapy. However, you won't be pressured to delve into the detailed aspects of the trauma right away. Exploring those moments is a gradual process that unfolds as trust and safety are established. The therapist's priority is to meet you where you are emotionally, ensuring that the space feels secure and respectful before diving into deeper discussions.

Setting Goals
You'll work with your therapist to establish goals for healing, whether that's improving communication, addressing emotional triggers, or rebuilding physical intimacy.

Exploring Trauma Together
Therapy provides a safe space to share your individual experiences and learn how trauma has affected each of you.

Your therapist may guide you through exercises to process the trauma, improve understanding, and develop empathy for each other's perspectives.

Building Coping Skills
You'll learn practical tools for managing stress, addressing emotional triggers, and supporting one another in the healing process.

Fostering Connection
Therapy will also focus on rebuilding trust, intimacy, and communication in your relationship, helping you move forward as a team.

Finding the Right Therapist

Choosing a therapist who understands birth trauma and its impact on relationships is crucial. Here are tips for finding the right fit:

Look for Trauma-Informed Care: Ensure the therapist has experience working with trauma and understands its effects on individuals and relationships.

Seek Recommendations: Ask for referrals from your healthcare provider, support groups, or trusted friends.

Ask Questions: During an initial consultation, ask about the therapist's experience with birth trauma and their approach to couples therapy.

Trust Your Instincts: The right therapist should make both you and your partner feel comfortable and supported.

The Partner's Role in Therapy

For the partner who did not give birth, therapy is an opportunity to share your perspective, address your own challenges, and learn how to better support your partner. Being actively involved in therapy demonstrates your commitment to healing together and ensures your voice is heard. Some partners worry that therapy will focus solely on the birthing person's trauma, but a good therapist will address the experiences and needs of both individuals.

***

Exercise: Preparing for Therapy

If you're considering therapy, this exercise will help you prepare for your first session and clarify your goals.

Step 1: Reflect Individually

Each partner takes 5-10 minutes to answer the following questions:

- What challenges or emotions have I been experiencing since the birth?
- How has trauma affected me personally and in my relationship?
- What do I hope to gain from therapy?

Step 2: Share Your Reflections

Take turns sharing your responses with each other. Use this as an opportunity to express your hopes and concerns about therapy.

Step 3: Identify Shared Goals

Together, discuss what you want to achieve as a couple. For example:

- "We want to feel more connected and communicate better."
- "We want to work through our fears and anxieties."

Step 4: Create a List of Questions

Write down any questions you have for the therapist, such as:

- "How do you approach couples therapy after birth trauma?"
- "What tools or strategies can we expect to learn?"

- "How can we involve both of our perspectives in the process?"

Therapy as a Catalyst for Healing

Therapy offers a unique and transformative opportunity for couples to address the deep and often unspoken impacts of birth trauma. It is not about assigning blame or "fixing" problems, but rather about creating a safe space where both partners can explore their experiences, emotions, and needs with the guidance of a skilled professional. The therapeutic process allows couples to uncover underlying issues, strengthen their connection, and work collaboratively toward healing and growth.

One of the most valuable aspects of therapy is the ability to approach trauma in a structured way. Birth trauma often leaves couples feeling overwhelmed, unsure of where to begin in their healing journey. A therapist helps break the process into manageable steps, guiding each partner in understanding their feelings, processing the trauma, and learning practical tools to rebuild their relationship. This structured approach creates a sense of progress, even when the journey feels daunting.

For many couples, therapy also provides validation for experiences that may have been dismissed or misunderstood elsewhere. Birth trauma is deeply personal, and it's common for both the birthing person and the partner to feel that their emotions are minimized or overlooked. A trauma-informed therapist acknowledges the unique challenges of birth trauma and creates an environment where each partner feels seen, heard, and respected. This validation can be profoundly healing, as it reminds both partners that their feelings and struggles are legitimate.

Therapy also acts as a bridge between partners, fostering empathy and understanding. Trauma often creates emotional distance, with each person processing their pain in isolation. Through guided conversations and exercises, therapy helps partners share their perspectives and develop a deeper appreciation for each other's experiences. This mutual understanding strengthens the relationship and lays the groundwork for rebuilding trust, intimacy, and connection.

Another key benefit of therapy is the opportunity to develop and practice coping strategies in a supportive environment. A therapist introduces tools for managing stress, navigating triggers, and improving communication, helping couples address the practical challenges of daily life after trauma. These strategies not only aid in the immediate healing process but also equip couples with skills they can use long after therapy ends.

For some couples, therapy is the first time they've prioritized their relationship since the trauma occurred. The arrival of a new baby, combined with the emotional weight of trauma, often leaves little time or energy for nurturing the partnership. By carving out dedicated time for therapy, couples signal their commitment to healing together. This intentional focus on their relationship can rekindle a sense of partnership and shared purpose.

Ultimately, therapy is a catalyst for healing because it empowers couples to confront their pain and move forward together. It transforms the trauma from something that divides into an experience that strengthens the bond between partners. While the process may be challenging, it is also deeply rewarding, as couples emerge with greater resilience, understanding, and connection.

Seeking professional help is not a sign of failure - it's a courageous and proactive step toward reclaiming your relationship and building a healthier, more fulfilling future. Therapy reminds couples that healing is possible, and it equips them with the tools and support they need to thrive in the face of adversity. By engaging in therapy, you're not only healing from the past—you're laying the foundation for a stronger, more connected partnership in the years to come.

Chapter 9
Creating a Support System

The Power of a Village

Healing from birth trauma can be an isolating experience, especially when it feels like no one truly understands what you've been through. However, the journey to recovery becomes more manageable - and often more meaningful - when you surround yourself with a strong support system. This "village" is not just a collection of people who help you with tasks; it's a network of individuals who listen, empathize, and share in your experiences without judgment. A well-built village provides emotional reassurance, practical assistance, and a sense of connection that can ease the weight of trauma.

For the birthing person, a village can offer invaluable emotional validation. After a traumatic birth, it's common to feel alone in your pain, as if no one else has experienced what you're going through. Supportive friends, family members, or peers remind you that your feelings are valid and that you don't have to carry the burden by yourself. Just having someone who listens without trying to "fix" the situation can make a world of difference, helping you process emotions that might otherwise feel overwhelming.

For the partner, a village can provide relief from the pressure of trying to be everything to everyone. Partners often feel like they need to hold it all together - supporting their loved one, caring for the baby, and managing household responsibilities. This can lead to emotional and physical burnout, leaving them with little energy to address their own needs. A support network lightens this load, allowing the partner to share caregiving responsibilities or find a listening ear for their own challenges.

A village also plays a crucial role in practical recovery. The demands of parenting are intense, and after a traumatic birth, these demands can feel even heavier. Supportive friends and family can step in to provide tangible help, such as preparing meals, running errands, or babysitting while you rest or attend therapy. These acts of service not only alleviate stress but also create space for you and your partner to focus on healing and bonding with your baby.

Beyond emotional and practical support, a village fosters a sense of belonging. Birth trauma can make you feel disconnected - not just from your partner, but from the world around you. Being surrounded by people who care reminds you that you're not alone. It strengthens your resilience and reinforces the idea that healing is a shared journey, one that doesn't have to be tackled in isolation. When you have a village, you're reminded that it's okay to lean on others, and that doing so doesn't make you weak - it makes you human.

Ultimately, the power of a village lies in its ability to remind you that healing does not have to be an individual journey. It's a communal effort, supported by those who care deeply about your well-being. With the right people in your corner, you'll feel more equipped to face the challenges of recovery and parenting, and more hopeful about the future you're building for yourself and your family.

Why Support Matters

Birth trauma can be isolating, especially when those around you don't fully understand what you've been through. A support system helps break that isolation by providing emotional validation, practical assistance, and a sense of connection. Support is not just about getting help with tasks - it's about having people who genuinely care about your well-being and are willing to stand beside you as you heal. For couples, a support network also provides relief from the pressures of parenting and caregiving, giving you the space to focus on your relationship and individual recovery.

Identifying Your Support Needs

Before building your support system, it's helpful to identify the areas where you need the most help. Consider these categories:

- **Emotional Support:** Someone who will listen without judgment and offer encouragement.
- **Practical Help:** Assistance with day-to-day tasks like cooking, cleaning, or running errands.
- **Parenting Support:** Guidance or help with caring for your baby, such as babysitting or advice from experienced parents.
- **Professional Support:** Access to therapists, counselors, or support groups specializing in trauma recovery.

By understanding your specific needs, you can seek out the right people and resources to fill those gaps.

Building Your Support Network

Creating a reliable support system may feel daunting, but it's a process that starts with small steps. Here's how to begin:

Reach Out to Trusted People

Start by identifying friends, family members, or colleagues who you feel comfortable opening up to. Choose individuals who are empathetic, dependable, and nonjudgmental.

Communicate Your Needs

Be clear about what kind of support you're seeking. For example:

- "I've been struggling emotionally since the birth and would love someone to talk to."
- "I'm feeling overwhelmed with household tasks and could use help with meal prep."

Join a Support Group

Look for local or online support groups for parents who have experienced birth trauma. These groups provide a sense of solidarity, allowing you to connect with others who truly understand your journey.

Utilize Professional Resources

Consider therapists, lactation consultants, doulas, or postpartum coaches who specialize in trauma recovery. Professional guidance can complement the emotional and practical support you receive from loved ones.

Accept Help When Offered

It can be hard to accept help, especially if you're used to being independent. Remind yourself that accepting support is not a sign of weakness - it's a step toward healing.

Involving Your Partner

A support system doesn't just benefit the birthing person; it's also vital for the partner. Partners often feel the pressure to "do it all" while supporting their loved one, which can lead to burnout. Encouraging your partner to seek their own sources of support - whether it's a friend, family member, or therapist - helps ensure they also have space to process their emotions and recharge.

Setting Boundaries with Support

While support is invaluable, it's also important to set boundaries. Not every offer of help will be aligned with your needs, and some well-meaning individuals may overstep. Here's how to navigate boundaries:

- Be honest about what's helpful versus what isn't. For example: "I appreciate your advice, but right now, I just need someone to listen."
- Politely decline offers that feel overwhelming. For instance: "Thank you for offering to visit, but we're focusing on quiet time at home this week."
- Protect your energy by limiting time with people who drain you emotionally or don't respect your healing process.

***

Exercise: Mapping Your Support System

This exercise helps you identify existing sources of support and highlight areas where you may need to seek additional help.

Step 1: Create a Support Map

Draw a circle in the center of a piece of paper and write your name or your family's name in the middle. Around the circle, create smaller circles for each source of support you currently have (e.g., partner, parent, friend, therapist).

Step 2: Assess Your Network

For each source of support, ask yourself:

- Are they meeting my emotional, practical, or parenting needs?
- Do I feel comfortable and safe with them?

Step 3: Identify Gaps

Notice any areas where you lack support. For example:

- Do you need more help with childcare?
- Are you missing someone to talk to about your emotions?

Step 4: Plan Next Steps
Write down one action you can take to fill each gap. Examples:

- Research local support groups.
- Ask a friend if they'd be willing to babysit once a week.
- Schedule a consultation with a trauma-informed therapist.

Healing Together with Support

Building a support system takes time, but the effort is worth it. Having people to lean on lightens the load and allows you to focus on what matters most - healing, bonding with your baby, and reconnecting as a couple. A strong network of support reinforces the idea that you don't have to face trauma alone. With the right people and resources by your side, you'll find strength in community and the encouragement to keep moving forward.

In the final chapter, we'll explore how to move forward as a team, celebrating the growth you've achieved and embracing the possibilities that lie ahead.

Chapter 10
Moving Forward as a Team

Healing as a Partnership

The journey through birth trauma can be deeply challenging, but it is also an opportunity to grow stronger as a couple. Moving forward as a team means navigating the complexities of trauma recovery, parenting, and rekindling your connection with intentionality and care. It's about finding ways to honor the pain you've endured while embracing the future with resilience, empathy, and shared purpose. This chapter focuses on reestablishing trust, intimacy, and a sense of normalcy, and celebrating the growth you've achieved as individuals and as partners.

Reestablishing Trust and Connection

Trauma can shake the foundation of trust in a relationship, even when neither partner is at fault. Rebuilding trust requires consistency, honesty, and vulnerability.

- **Consistency Over Time**: Trust grows when both partners show up for each other consistently, even in small ways. Whether it's honoring commitments, being emotionally present, or simply checking in daily, these actions help rebuild a sense of reliability and safety.
- **Open Communication**: Share your thoughts, fears, and hopes with one another regularly. Being transparent about your feelings fosters a deeper connection and helps prevent misunderstandings.
- **Vulnerability and Empathy**: Healing requires both partners to be vulnerable. By expressing your emotions honestly and listening to each other with empathy, you create an environment where trust can flourish.

Rediscovering Intimacy

For many couples, intimacy feels distant after birth trauma, both emotionally and physically. Moving forward as a team means rekindling that closeness in ways that feel safe and comfortable for both partners.

- **Start Small**: Intimacy doesn't have to begin with sex. Simple gestures like holding hands, cuddling, or making eye contact can help rebuild physical connection.
- **Prioritize Emotional Closeness**: Emotional intimacy is the foundation of physical closeness. Spend time talking, laughing, or enjoying shared activities to nurture your bond.
- **Take It at Your Own Pace**: There's no "right" timeline for restoring intimacy. Honor each other's boundaries and communicate openly about what feels comfortable.

Creating a "New Normal"

Life after trauma is rarely the same as it was before, but that doesn't mean it can't be fulfilling. Moving forward involves embracing a "new normal" that reflects the growth and changes you've experienced.

- **Define Your Priorities**: Discuss what matters most to you as a couple and as a family. Whether it's quality time together, shared parenting goals, or personal growth, aligning on priorities helps create a sense of purpose.
- **Simplify Where You Can**: Let go of unrealistic expectations or unnecessary obligations. Focus your energy on what truly supports your healing and connection.
- **Celebrate Progress**: Take time to acknowledge how far you've come. Whether it's overcoming a specific challenge or simply surviving a difficult week, every step forward is worth celebrating.

Building Resilience Together

Resilience is the ability to adapt and thrive in the face of adversity. Birth trauma may have tested your relationship, but it also offers an opportunity to develop greater strength and understanding as a couple.

- **Lean on Each Other**: View yourselves as a team tackling challenges together, rather than as individuals facing separate battles. This perspective fosters unity and mutual support.
- **Learn from the Experience**: Reflect on what the trauma has taught you about yourselves, each other, and your relationship. Use these insights to strengthen your bond.
- **Embrace Flexibility**: Life is unpredictable, and healing doesn't follow a straight line. Be willing to adjust your plans and expectations as needed, and approach setbacks with patience.

Celebrating Your Growth

While the pain of trauma may never fully disappear, it doesn't have to overshadow the progress you've made. Take time to recognize the ways you've grown as individuals and as a couple.

- **Celebrate Your Resilience**: Surviving and healing from trauma is an achievement in itself. Acknowledge the strength and determination it took to reach this point.
- **Honor Your Partnership**: Reflect on how you've supported each other through difficult times. Whether it's through small gestures or significant sacrifices, these efforts are the foundation of your relationship.
- **Focus on the Future**: While it's important to honor the past, allow yourselves to look forward with hope and excitement. Consider what kind of future you want to build together and take steps toward making it a reality.

***

Exercise: Visioning Your Future Together

This exercise helps you and your partner align on your shared vision for the future and create actionable steps to move forward as a team.

Step 1: Reflect Individually

Take 10 minutes to write down your thoughts on the following questions:

- What do I hope for our relationship in the next year?
- What strengths have we developed as a couple that I want to continue building on?
- What areas do I think we need to work on together?

Step 2: Share Your Reflections

Take turns sharing your answers with each other. Focus on listening and understanding rather than critiquing or solving.

Step 3: Define Shared Goals

Together, identify 2-3 goals for your relationship or family in the coming months. Examples:

- "Spend one evening a week focused on connecting as a couple."
- "Work on better communicating our needs."
- "Plan a family outing once a month to create joyful memories."

Step 4: Create Actionable Steps

For each goal, outline one small step you can take this week to move closer to it. For example:

- For communication: "Schedule a weekly check-in to talk about our feelings."
- For connection: "Plan a date night at home this Friday."

Moving Forward with Hope

Moving forward after birth trauma is not about erasing the past but about embracing the future with strength and intention. By prioritizing healing, nurturing your relationship, and celebrating your growth, you can build a life filled with love, connection, and resilience. Together, you've faced profound challenges - and together, you have the capacity to create a beautiful, fulfilling future.

Healing as a team is an ongoing process, but it's also a rewarding one. Each step you take brings you closer to a stronger, more united partnership. This journey has been one of resilience, and the next chapters of your life are yours to shape - together.

Notes

68

Notes

Notes

Notes

71

Notes

Notes

Notes

Notes

75